DIVINE HEALTH AFFIRMATIONS AGAINST HEART FAILURE

.....A Therapy that Works....

BY
IHEKE WILLIAMS

COPYRIGHT © 2019, IHEKE WILLIAMS

Unless otherwise indicated, all scripture quotations are taken from the King James Version of the Bible
A key for other Bible versions used

NKJV	New King James Version
AMP	The Amplified Bible
TANT	The New Amplified Bible
TLB -	The Living Bible
CEV -	Contemporary English Version
NASB	New American Standard Version
GW -	God's Word version
ESV -	English Standard Version
NET -	New English Translation
ISV -	International Standard Version
NIV -	New International Version
MSG -	The Message Translation

<u>DEDICATION</u>

This Book is dedicated to Almighty God and to everyone in the world.

TABLE OF CONTENT

WHAT IS HEART FAILURE?

Cardiovascular disease (**CVD**) is a class of diseases that involve the heart or blood vessels. CVD includes coronary artery diseases(CAD) such as angina and myocardial infarction (commonly known as a heart attack).

Other CVDs include stroke, heart failure, hypertensive heart disease, rheumatic heart disease, cardiomyopathy, heart arrhythmia, congenital heart disease, valvular heart disease, carditis, aortic aneurysms, peripheral artery disease, thromboembolic disease, and venous thrombosis.

Source: Wikipedia

WHAT IS GOD'S SOLUTION

"...By His wounds ye have been healed.."
1 Peter 2:24

JESUS has already healed you over 2000 years ago.

Your heart is Active, Strong and Perfect Forever because of the wound Jesus suffered on the cross for your sake.

You have NO business with heart failure or a weak heart.

For the next 31 days, you will affirm this blessing in your life and you will live with a perfectly functioning heart forever.

INSTRUCTION 1

That if thou shalt confess with thy mouth the Lord Jesus, and shalt believe in thine heart that God hath raised him from the dead, thou shalt be saved. – Romans 10:9

There has to be a connection with what you say and what you have in your heart. We believe with our heart, this is the reason you have to meditate on the gospel with your heart, believe it and then affirm it.

For the affirmations to be effective, you will have to meditate on the scripture (1Peter 2:24) for 5 minutes, in your heart, and then affirm it.

INSTRUCTION 2

"For our light affliction, which is but for a moment, worketh for us a far more exceeding and eternal weight of glory;

While we look NOT at the things which are seen, but at the things which are not seen: for the things which are seen are temporal; but the things which are not seen are eternal. –
2 Corinthians 4:17-18

Do not touch any part of your body that has been affected by this disease for the duration of the affirmations.

Follow these instructions and your affirmations will be effective.

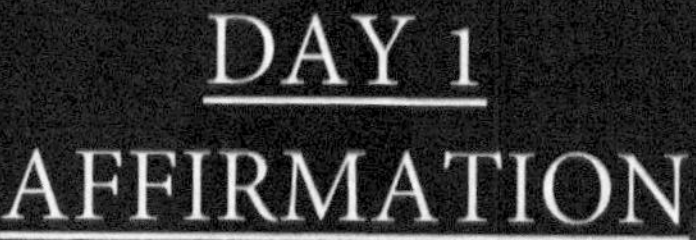

DAY 1
AFFIRMATION

Meditate on 1 Peter 2:24B in your heart for 5 minutes
"..By His stripes ye have been healed.."

Now Affirm the Blessing

"I HAVE BEEN HEALED THEREFORE, I AFFIRM THAT MY HEART IS NOT WEAK!"

DAY 2
AFFIRMATION

Meditate on 1 Peter 2:24B in your
heart for 5 minutes
" ..By His stripes ye have been
healed.."

Now Affirm the Blessing

"I HAVE BEEN HEALED THEREFORE, I AFFIRM THAT MY HEART DOES NOT FAIL !"

DAY 3
AFFIRMATION

Meditate on 1 Peter 2:24B in your heart for 5 minutes
"..By His stripes ye have been healed.."

Now Affirm the Blessing

"I HAVE BEEN HEALED THEREFORE, I AFFIRM THAT MY HEART IS ACTIVE AND PERFECT FOREVER!"

DAY 4
AFFIRMATION

Meditate on 1 Peter 2:24B in your
heart for 5 minutes
"..By His stripes ye have been
healed.."

Now Affirm the Blessing

**"I HAVE BEEN HEALED
THEREFORE, I AFFIRM
THAT MY HEART IS
ACTIVE AND PERFECT
FOREVER!"**

DAY 5
AFFIRMATION

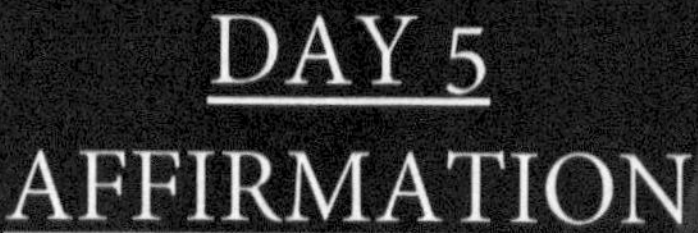

Meditate on 1 Peter 2:24B in your
heart for 5 minutes
"..By His stripes ye have been
healed.."

Now Affirm the Blessing

"I HAVE BEEN HEALED THEREFORE, I AFFIRM THAT MY HEART IS ACTIVE AND PERFECT FOREVER!"

DAY 6
AFFIRMATION

Meditate on 1 Peter 2:24B in your
heart for 5 minutes
"..By His stripes ye have been
healed.."

Now Affirm the Blessing

**"I HAVE BEEN HEALED
THEREFORE, I AFFIRM
THAT MY HEART IS
ACTIVE AND PERFECT
FOREVER!"**

DAY 7
AFFIRMATION

Meditate on 1 Peter 2:24B in your heart for 5 minutes
"..By His stripes ye have been healed.."

Now Affirm the Blessing

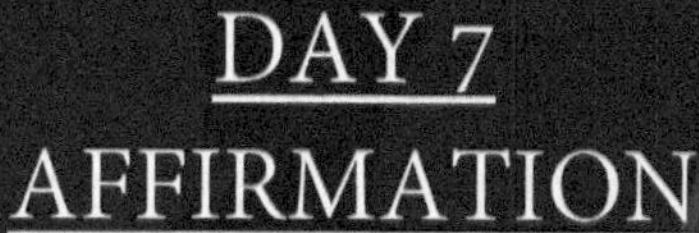

"I HAVE BEEN HEALED THEREFORE, I AFFIRM THAT MY HEART IS ACTIVE AND PERFECT FOREVER!"

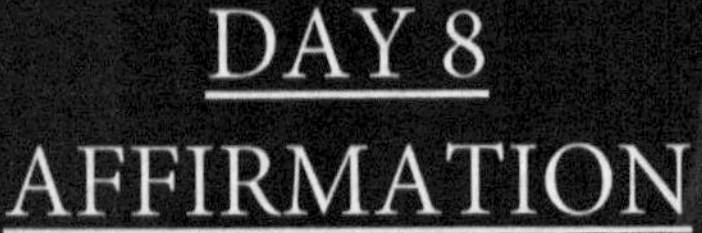

DAY 8
AFFIRMATION

Meditate on 1 Peter 2:24B in your
heart for 5 minutes
"..By His stripes ye have been
healed.."

Now Affirm the Blessing

"I HAVE BEEN HEALED
THEREFORE, I AFFIRM
THAT MY HEART IS
ACTIVE AND PERFECT
FOREVER!"

DAY 9
AFFIRMATION

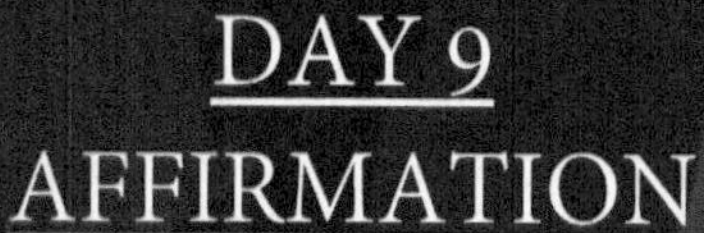

Meditate on 1 Peter 2:24B in your
heart for 5 minutes
"..By His stripes ye have been
healed.."

Now Affirm the Blessing

"I HAVE BEEN HEALED THEREFORE, I AFFIRM THAT MY HEART IS ACTIVE AND PERFECT FOREVER!"

DAY 10
AFFIRMATION

Meditate on 1 Peter 2:24B in your
heart for 5 minutes
"..By His stripes ye have been
healed.."

Now Affirm the Blessing

"I HAVE BEEN HEALED THEREFORE, I AFFIRM THAT MY HEART IS ACTIVE AND PERFECT FOREVER!"

DAY 11
AFFIRMATION

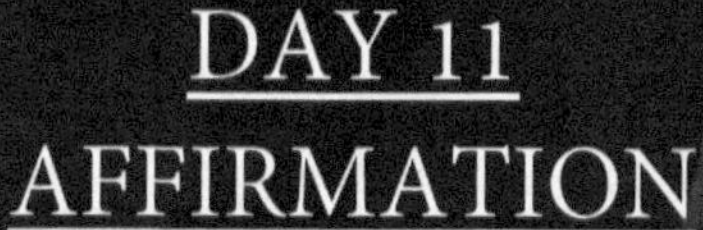

Meditate on 1 Peter 2:24B in your heart for 5 minutes
"..By His stripes ye have been healed.."

Now Affirm the Blessing

"I HAVE BEEN HEALED THEREFORE, I AFFIRM THAT MY HEART IS ACTIVE AND PERFECT FOREVER!"

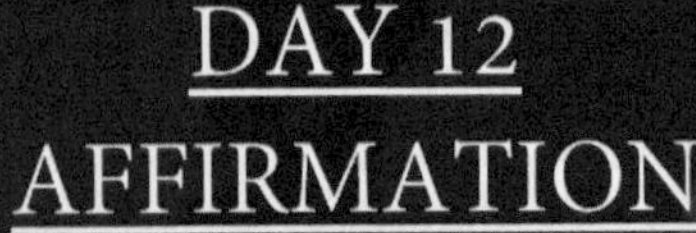

DAY 12
AFFIRMATION

Meditate on 1 Peter 2:24B in your
heart for 5 minutes
"..By His stripes ye have been
healed.."

Now Affirm the Blessing

"I HAVE BEEN HEALED
THEREFORE, I AFFIRM
THAT MY HEART IS
ACTIVE AND PERFECT
FOREVER!"

DAY 13
AFFIRMATION

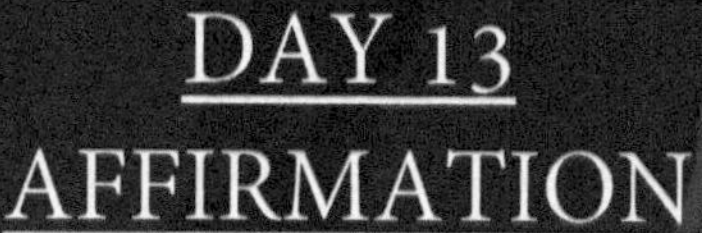

Meditate on 1 Peter 2:24B in your
heart for 5 minutes
"..By His stripes ye have been
healed.."

Now Affirm the Blessing

"I HAVE BEEN HEALED THEREFORE, I AFFIRM THAT MY HEART IS ACTIVE AND PERFECT FOREVER!"

DAY 14
AFFIRMATION

Meditate on 1 Peter 2:24B in your
heart for 5 minutes
" ..By His stripes ye have been
healed.."

Now Affirm the Blessing

"I HAVE BEEN HEALED THEREFORE, I AFFIRM THAT MY HEART IS ACTIVE AND PERFECT FOREVER!"

DAY 15
AFFIRMATION

Meditate on 1 Peter 2:24B in your heart for 5 minutes

"..By His stripes ye have been healed.."

Now Affirm the Blessing

"I HAVE BEEN HEALED THEREFORE, I AFFIRM THAT MY HEART IS ACTIVE AND PERFECT FOREVER!"

DAY 16
AFFIRMATION

Meditate on 1 Peter 2:24B in your
heart for 5 minutes
"..By His stripes ye have been
healed.."

Now Affirm the Blessing

"I HAVE BEEN HEALED THEREFORE, I AFFIRM THAT MY HEART IS ACTIVE AND PERFECT FOREVER!"

DAY 17
AFFIRMATION

Meditate on 1 Peter 2:24B in your
heart for 5 minutes
"..By His stripes ye have been
healed.."

Now Affirm the Blessing

"I HAVE BEEN HEALED THEREFORE, I AFFIRM THAT MY HEART IS ACTIVE AND PERFECT FOREVER!"

DAY 18
AFFIRMATION

Meditate on 1 Peter 2:24B in your
heart for 5 minutes
"..By His stripes ye have been
healed.."

Now Affirm the Blessing

"I HAVE BEEN HEALED THEREFORE, I AFFIRM THAT MY HEART IS ACTIVE AND PERFECT FOREVER!"

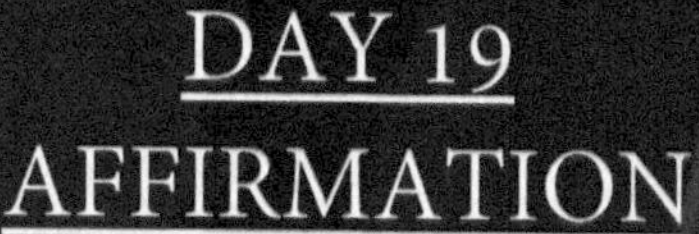

DAY 19
AFFIRMATION

Meditate on 1 Peter 2:24B in your
heart for 5 minutes
"..By His stripes ye have been
healed.."

Now Affirm the Blessing

"I HAVE BEEN HEALED
THEREFORE, I AFFIRM
THAT MY HEART IS
ACTIVE AND PERFECT
FOREVER!"

DAY 20
AFFIRMATION

Meditate on 1 Peter 2:24B in your
heart for 5 minutes
"..By His stripes ye have been
healed.."

Now Affirm the Blessing

"I HAVE BEEN HEALED THEREFORE, I AFFIRM THAT MY HEART IS ACTIVE AND PERFECT FOREVER!"

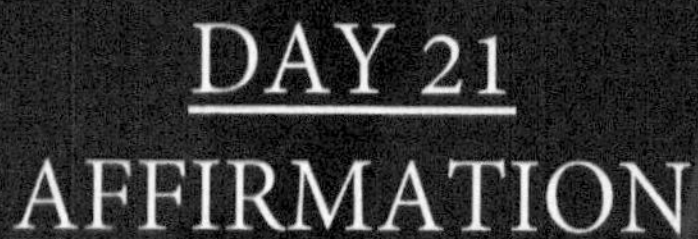

DAY 21
AFFIRMATION

Meditate on 1 Peter 2:24B in your
heart for 5 minutes
"..By His stripes ye have been
healed.."

Now Affirm the Blessing

"I HAVE BEEN HEALED THEREFORE, I AFFIRM THAT MY HEART IS ACTIVE AND PERFECT FOREVER!"

DAY 22
AFFIRMATION

Meditate on 1 Peter 2:24B in your heart for 5 minutes
"..By His stripes ye have been healed.."

Now Affirm the Blessing

"I HAVE BEEN HEALED THEREFORE, I AFFIRM THAT MY HEART IS ACTIVE AND PERFECT FOREVER!"

DAY 23
AFFIRMATION

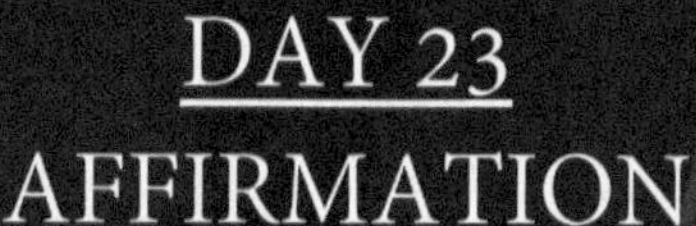

Meditate on 1 Peter 2:24B in your
heart for 5 minutes
"..By His stripes ye have been
healed.."

Now Affirm the Blessing

"I HAVE BEEN HEALED
THEREFORE, I AFFIRM
THAT MY HEART IS
ACTIVE AND PERFECT
FOREVER!"

DAY 24
AFFIRMATION

Meditate on 1 Peter 2:24B in your
heart for 5 minutes
"..By His stripes ye have been
healed.."

Now Affirm the Blessing

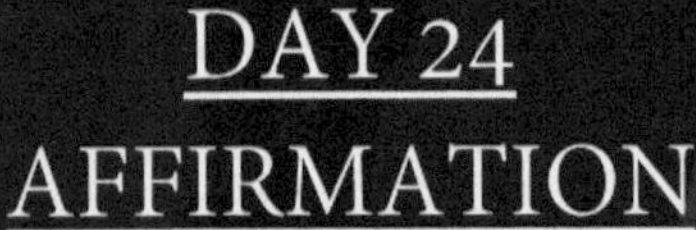

**"I HAVE BEEN HEALED
THEREFORE, I AFFIRM
THAT MY HEART IS
ACTIVE AND PERFECT
FOREVER!"**

DAY 25
AFFIRMATION

Meditate on 1 Peter 2:24B in your
heart for 5 minutes
"..By His stripes ye have been
healed.."

Now Affirm the Blessing

"I HAVE BEEN HEALED THEREFORE, I AFFIRM THAT MY HEART IS ACTIVE AND PERFECT FOREVER!"

DAY 26
AFFIRMATION

Meditate on 1 Peter 2:24B in your
heart for 5 minutes
"..By His stripes ye have been
healed.."

Now Affirm the Blessing

"I HAVE BEEN HEALED THEREFORE, I AFFIRM THAT MY HEART IS ACTIVE AND PERFECT FOREVER!"

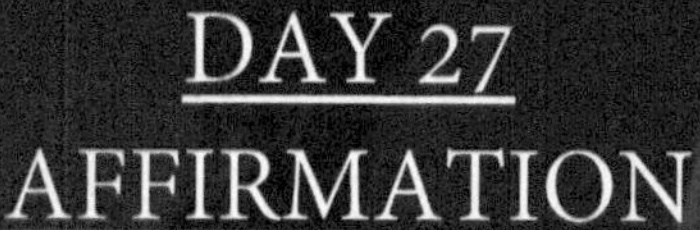

DAY 27
AFFIRMATION

Meditate on 1 Peter 2:24B in your
heart for 5 minutes
"..By His stripes ye have been
healed.."

Now Affirm the Blessing

"I HAVE BEEN HEALED
THEREFORE, I AFFIRM
THAT MY HEART IS
ACTIVE AND PERFECT
FOREVER!"

DAY 28
AFFIRMATION

Meditate on 1 Peter 2:24B in your
heart for 5 minutes
"..By His stripes ye have been
healed.."

Now Affirm the Blessing

"I HAVE BEEN HEALED THEREFORE, I AFFIRM THAT MY HEART IS ACTIVE AND PERFECT FOREVER!"

DAY 29
AFFIRMATION

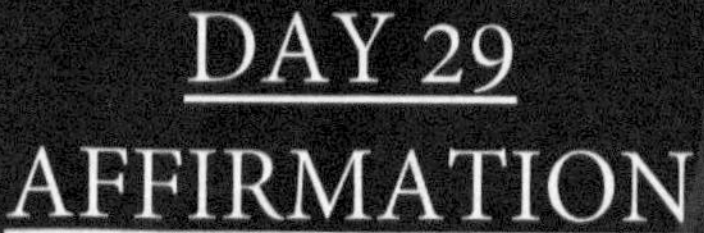

Meditate on 1 Peter 2:24B in your
heart for 5 minutes
"..By His stripes ye have been
healed.."

Now Affirm the Blessing

"I HAVE BEEN HEALED THEREFORE, I AFFIRM THAT MY HEART IS ACTIVE AND PERFECT FOREVER!"

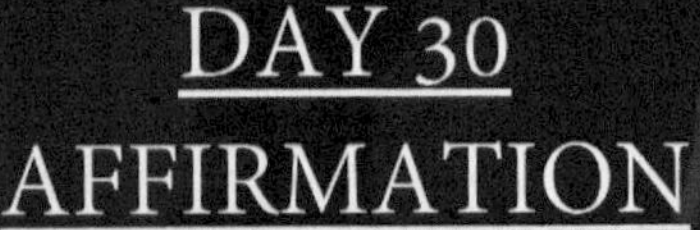

DAY 30
AFFIRMATION

Meditate on 1 Peter 2:24B in your
heart for 5 minutes
"..By His stripes ye have been
healed.."

Now Affirm the Blessing

"I HAVE BEEN HEALED
THEREFORE, I AFFIRM
THAT MY HEART IS
ACTIVE AND PERFECT
FOREVER!"

DAY 31
AFFIRMATION

Meditate on 1 Peter 2:24B in your
heart for 5 minutes
"..By His stripes ye have been
healed.."

Now Affirm the Blessing

"I HAVE BEEN HEALED THEREFORE, I AFFIRM THAT MY HEART IS ACTIVE AND PERFECT FOREVER!"

SUMMARY

1 Peter 2:24
"..By His stripes ye have been healed.."

Heart failure does not exist in you. Our Lord JESUS Christ has healed you already.

YOUR HEART IS ACTIVE, STRONG AND WORKING PERFECTLY FOREVER!!!

Rejoice and live in Divine Health all the days of your life.

PRAYER FOR SALVATION

We believe that you have been blessed and that you want to receive eternal life that God has made available to everyone who believes in his love and his grace which He expressed lavishly through His Son Jesus Christ.

"For God so loved the world, that He gave his only begotten Son, that whosoever believeth in him should not perish, but have everlasting life." - John 3:16

Say this prayer to God and believe it with your heart

"Father, I believe that you gave me your only Son to die for my sin. I believe you raised Him from the dead. I declare that your son, Jesus Christ is the Lord of my life. I receive eternal life and I receive the Holy Spirit. I am saved forever.in Jesus name. I am so Happy that today and forever, I am your child. Amen ".

Congratulations, you are now a child of God Halleluyah!! – John 1:12

OTHER INFORMATION

Please share your testimonies via the following handles;

<ihekewilliams@gmail.com>
+2348061530541

Other Books written by the author includes
Dad, Pray for your Daughter
Mum, Pray for your Daughter
Mum, pray for your Son
Don't stop the flow of the Blessing
Daddy's Prayers
Mummy's Prayers
Divine Health Affirmation Against Cancer
Divine Health Affirmation Against Atshma
Divine Health Affirmation Against Malaria
Divine Health Affirmation Series

ABOUT THE AUTHOR

Iheke Williams is a firm follower and disciple of the Lord Jesus Christ. He is a passionate minister of the grace of our Lord and savior Jesus Christ and has brought the reality of the divine life of Christ into the lives of so many.

Iheke Williams has a calling to communicate the gospel of Christ with simplicity and to show the world how to activate the eternal life of God that is in us already which includes Divine health, Divine righteousness, Divine security and Divine prosperity.

As you read this book and other books written by Iheke Williams you will literally begin to function and manifest the life of God that is already inside you to the glory of God the Father who is the author of all grace and mercy. Amen.

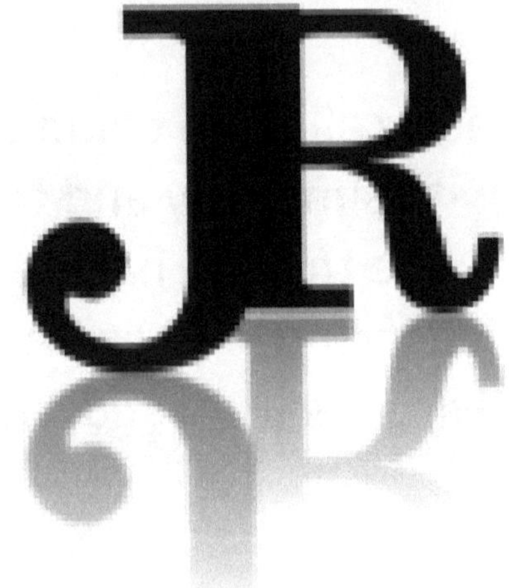

www.ingramcontent.com/pod-product-compliance
Lightning Source LLC
Chambersburg PA
CBHW051425250726

48655CB00003B/1235